A Practical Approach
to
Life After Yeast Infection

Jaylen Fleming

form or by any means, including photocopying, recording, or other electronic or mechanical methods, without the prior written permission of the publisher, except in the case of brief quotations embodied in critical reviews and certain other noncommercial uses permitted by copyright law.

Table of Contents

About the Author

Hi, I am Dr. Jaylen Fleming. With over 10 years of clinical experience, I am a seasoned publisher, dedicated to providing compassionate self-help resources on human health issues and diseases to patients and other health practitioners. Follow me for updates, and get my books to keep yourself enlightened and liberated.

Other books by same Author

- Post Sepsis Syndrome: PSS Management Guide - Jaylen Fleming
- Post Sepsis Syndrome: Health after Sepsis,Healing after Sepsis -Jaylen Fleming

- Septic Shock - Jaylen Fleming
- Sarah's Battle -Jaylen Fleming
- Sepsis Symptoms Handbook -Jaylen Fleming
- Post Angelman Syndrome - Jaylen Fleming
- Post Tourette Syndrome - Jaylen Fleming

<u>LIFE AFTER SEPSIS</u>

According to a recent report, approximately half of patients who survived a hospitalization for sepsis often have incomplete recovery. This book is a guide to help sepsis survivors manage **"POST SEPSIS SYNDROME"** - Look inside for more detail .

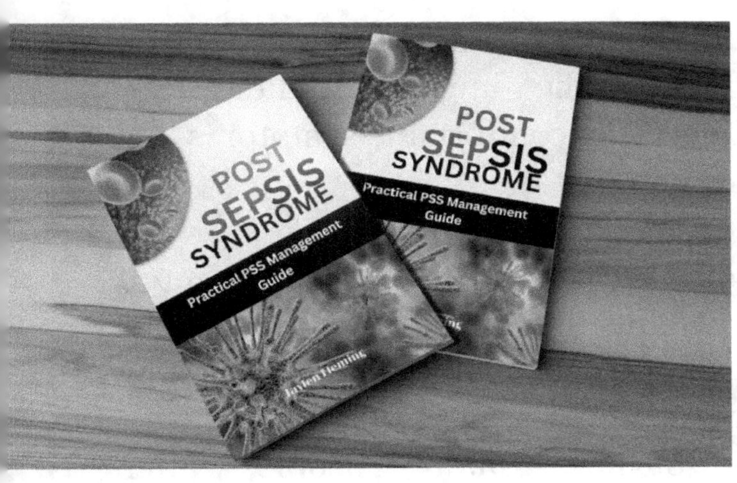

Introduction

Yeast infections are an incredibly common yet often misunderstood condition that affects millions of people, primarily women, but also men and children. Despite their prevalence, many individuals suffer in silence, embarrassed to discuss their symptoms or unaware that what they're experiencing is treatable. Yeast infections, caused by an overgrowth of the fungus *Candida*, can disrupt daily life with uncomfortable symptoms like itching, burning, and irritation.

However, life after a yeast infection is about more than just overcoming these symptoms. It's about regaining control of your body, understanding how to prevent future infections, and finding peace with your health journey. Many people, after experiencing recurrent yeast infections, feel frustrated or defeated. They may wonder why it keeps happening, what they're doing wrong, and how they can stop the cycle. This book is designed to answer those questions and more.

In **"A Practical Approach to Life After Yeast Infection,"** we will explore not only the medical side of yeast infections but also the emotional and mental toll they can take. You'll learn how to heal physically, prevent future infections, and approach life with a renewed sense of confidence and well-being. Whether you've dealt with one yeast infection or recurrent ones, this book will guide you through the process of reclaiming your health.

Chapter One

Your Body After Yeast Infections

After experiencing a yeast infection, your body goes through a process of healing and recovery. While the infection may be resolved, the aftermath can leave lingering effects that are important to address. Understanding how yeast infections affect different parts of your body helps in fully recovering and preventing future issues.

How Yeast Infections Affect Your Body

A yeast infection, primarily caused by *Candida albicans*, impacts various areas of the body. The most commonly affected regions are the vaginal area in women and the skin, mouth, or digestive tract in others. These infections occur when the natural balance of microorganisms in your body is disrupted, leading to an overgrowth of yeast.

Here's how yeast infections typically affect your body:
- Vaginal area: In women, yeast infections can cause intense itching, burning, and irritation, making daily activities uncomfortable. Swelling, redness, and a thick, white discharge are also common symptoms.
- Skin: For those experiencing yeast infections in skin folds (e.g., under the breasts, groin, or armpits), redness, soreness, and rash can occur.

- Mouth (Oral Thrush): White patches in the mouth or throat, soreness, and difficulty swallowing are signs of yeast overgrowth in the oral cavity.
- Digestive Tract: When yeast overgrowth occurs in the gut, it can cause bloating, gas, and digestive discomfort.

While these symptoms typically resolve after treatment, it's essential to recognize that your body may need time to fully recover.

Physical Recovery and Healing

After a yeast infection, your body's natural balance needs to be restored. Even though antifungal treatments help eliminate the overgrowth, it's crucial to support your body in rebuilding its defenses.

- Rehydration and Skin Recovery: If the skin was affected, gentle skincare is necessary. Avoid using harsh soaps or irritants on affected areas. Instead, opt for mild, fragrance-free cleansers, and keep the area dry and clean.

- Gut Health Restoration: Since yeast overgrowth can disrupt the balance of good bacteria in your gut, supporting your digestive system with probiotics and a healthy diet is key. Fermented foods like yogurt, kefir, and sauerkraut can help reintroduce beneficial bacteria into your system, aiding recovery.

- Boosting Immunity: Strengthening your immune system can also help prevent recurrent infections. Eating a balanced diet rich in vitamins and antioxidants (especially Vitamin C, zinc, and probiotics) will improve your body's ability to fight off future infections.

Impact on Immune System and Gut Health

Yeast infections, especially recurring ones, can indicate underlying imbalances in your immune system or gut health. Your body's microbiome—composed of various bacteria and yeast—plays a rucial role in keeping these infections in check. When this balance is disrupted, yeast can thrive, leading to frequent infections.

Immune Response: If your immune system is weakened, you're more susceptible to yeast infections. Conditions like diabetes, autoimmune diseases, or even high stress levels can weaken your immune defenses, making it harder to fight off infections. After a yeast infection, it's important to focus on lifestyle changes that boost immunity, such as regular exercise, proper sleep, and stress management.

- Gut Health Connection: The health of your digestive tract plays a significant role in yeast overgrowth. A healthy gut is packed with good bacteria that prevent yeast from multiplying uncontrollably. However, factors like antibiotic use, poor diet, and chronic stress can reduce these good bacteria and allow yeast to flourish. Restoring gut health after a yeast infection is vital for preventing recurrences.

Long-Term Effects and Prevention

While most yeast infections are manageable and treatable, recurrent infections can signal a more persistent issue, such as chronic imbalances in the body. If left untreated or ignored, repeated infections can lead to skin damage, persistent irritation, and even emotional stress.

- Vaginal Health Maintenance: After a yeast infection, it's essential to maintain a healthy vaginal pH. Avoiding scented products, douching, and wearing breathable fabrics like cotton can help reduce irritation and maintain balance.
- Hygiene and Self-Care: Regular hygiene practices and paying attention to your body's signals are key to preventing future infections. Keeping areas prone to infection dry, wearing loose-fitting clothes, and using moisture-wicking fabrics can help minimize risk.

Chapter Two

Overcoming the Stigma of Chronic Yeast Infections

Living with chronic yeast infections can be frustrating, not only because of the physical discomfort but also because of the stigma that surrounds it. Many people who suffer from recurring yeast infections feel embarrassed or ashamed, which can lead to feelings of isolation. However, it's important to remember that yeast infections are a common medical condition, and there's no shame in seeking help or discussing it openly.

Understanding the Stigma

Yeast infections, particularly when chronic, are often surrounded by misinformation and misconceptions. Many associate the condition with poor hygiene or sexual behavior, which can contribute to the shame people feel. In reality, chronic yeast infections can be caused by a range of factors, including hormonal imbalances, immune system issues, or even frequent use of antibiotics.

For women, the stigma is often heightened by cultural expectations of feminine hygiene and purity. A recurring infection might make someone feel like they've failed to take care of their body or that their condition is somehow abnormal. This couldn't be further from the truth—yeast infections affect millions of people every year, and they have little to do with personal hygiene or morality.

Breaking the Silence

One of the most powerful ways to combat the stigma surrounding chronic yeast infections is to talk about them openly. Whether it's with a healthcare provider, a friend, or a support group, breaking the silence helps to normalize the conversation and dismantle the shame associated with the condition.

- Talking to Your Doctor: Chronic yeast infections can be a complex condition, so it's essential to have open and honest communication with your healthcare provider. Share your concerns, symptoms, and frustrations without hesitation. The more information your doctor has, the better they can tailor a treatment plan that works for you.

- Opening Up to Loved Ones: Talking about yeast infections with friends or family may seem uncomfortable, but sharing your experiences can be liberating. It's a way to let go of the guilt and secrecy that often surrounds the condition. You might even discover that others in your life have dealt with similar issues and can offer advice or support.

- Seeking Support Groups: Many people find comfort in joining communities where they can connect with others who have gone through the same experiences. Online forums, social media groups, and even local support groups can offer a safe space to share frustrations, learn new coping strategies, and feel less alone in the journey.

Educating Yourself and Others

Another key way to overcome the stigma is through education—both for yourself and for those around you. By understanding the true causes of yeast infections and how common they are, you can shift the narrative from shame to empowerment.

Know the Facts: Chronic yeast infections aren't a reflection of poor hygiene or improper self-care. They can occur for a variety of reasons, such as imbalances in the microbiome, hormonal shifts, or immune system weaknesses. Understanding the underlying causes can help you respond to the condition without self-blame.

Informing Others: If someone in your life perpetuates the stigma by making uninformed comments or jokes, use it as an opportunity to educate them. Let them know that yeast infections are a medical condition that can happen to anyone. By spreading accurate information, you contribute to breaking down the stigma for everyone.

Building Emotional Resilience

Living with a chronic condition like recurring yeast infections can take a toll on your mental and emotional health. Dealing with the physical symptoms, along with the social stigma, can lead to feelings of anxiety, frustration, and even depression. Building emotional resilience is essential for managing these challenges.

- Practice Self-Compassion: It's easy to fall into negative self-talk when you're dealing with chronic yeast infections. You might feel like your body is betraying you or that you're somehow at fault. Practicing self-compassion means acknowledging that you're doing your best to manage a condition that's beyond your control. Be kind to yourself and recognize that you deserve care and support, just like anyone else.

- Mindfulness and Stress Reduction: Chronic infections can be exacerbated by stress, so finding ways to manage stress is crucial. Mindfulness techniques like meditation, yoga, or deep breathing can help you stay grounded and reduce the mental burden of dealing with recurrent infections.

- Seeking Professional Help: If the emotional weight of dealing with chronic yeast infections becomes too much, don't hesitate to seek professional support. A therapist or counselor can help you navigate the emotions associated with chronic illness and develop coping strategies for managing the stigma and stress.

Reclaiming Your Confidence

Finally, it's essential to reclaim your sense of confidence and agency over your body. Living with a chronic condition like recurring yeast infections doesn't define you. By taking proactive steps to manage your health and challenging the stigma surrounding the condition, you can move forward with confidence.

- Focus on What You Can Control: While you may not be able to prevent every future yeast infection, you can take control of how you manage your health. Building habits that support your body's natural balance—like maintaining a healthy diet, managing stress, and seeking medical advice when needed—can help you feel empowered.

- Redefining Intimacy: Chronic yeast infections can affect your relationships and intimacy, but they don't have to define them. Open communication with your partner, understanding your body's needs, and giving yourself time to heal can strengthen your sense of self-worth and intimacy.

Chapter Three

Rebuilding Your Health

After battling a yeast infection, especially if it's been a recurring issue, your body needs time and attention to fully recover. Rebuilding your health involves taking a holistic approach that includes diet, lifestyle changes, and boosting your immune system to help your body restore its natural balance. This chapter will guide you through practical steps to strengthen your body and prevent future infections.

Dietary Changes for Long-term Wellness

Your diet plays a crucial role in maintaining the balance of good bacteria and yeast in your body, particularly in your gut and vaginal microbiome. Certain foods can either promote yeast growth or help to inhibit it, so making thoughtful dietary choices can aid in both recovery and prevention.

- Reduce Sugar and Refined Carbohydrates: Yeast thrives on sugar, so one of the most effective ways to prevent its overgrowth is by cutting down on sugary foods, processed snacks, and refined carbohydrates like white bread and pasta. Instead, focus on whole grains, vegetables, and healthy sources of protein.

- Incorporate More Fiber: A diet rich in fiber helps to maintain a healthy gut environment by promoting regular digestion and supporting the growth of good bacteria. Fiber-rich foods like fruits, vegetables, legumes, and whole grains can help improve gut health, making it harder for yeast to proliferate.

- Limit Dairy and Alcohol: Both dairy products and alcohol can contribute to yeast overgrowth in some individuals. While not everyone needs to eliminate these completely, cutting back on them may help reduce the risk of recurrent infections.

Probiotics and Supplements: What Helps?

One of the key strategies for rebuilding your health after a yeast infection is to support your body's natural defenses with probiotics and specific supplements. Probiotics help replenish the good bacteria in your gut and vaginal area, which can prevent yeast from growing out of control.

- Probiotics: These are beneficial bacteria that support a healthy microbiome. Probiotic supplements that contain strains like *Lactobacillus acidophilus* can help restore balance in the body. You can also add probiotic-rich foods to your diet, such as yogurt, kefir, sauerkraut, and kimchi.

Prebiotics: These are the fibers that feed good bacteria and help them flourish. Foods like garlic, onions, bananas, and asparagus are good sources of prebiotics that promote a healthy microbiome.

Antifungal Supplements: Certain natural supplements, such as oregano oil, garlic extract, and caprylic acid, have antifungal properties that can help control yeast overgrowth. These should be used under the guidance of a healthcare professional to ensure safe and effective use.

- Vitamins and Minerals: Supporting your immune system with a range of vitamins and minerals is essential. Vitamin C, vitamin D, zinc, and B-complex vitamins all play a role in immune function, and maintaining healthy levels can help your body fend off infections.

Exercise and Lifestyle Modifications

In addition to diet and supplements, making certain lifestyle changes can significantly impact your recovery and overall health. Regular physical activity and stress management play a vital role in reducing the risk of future yeast infections.

- Regular Exercise: Physical activity helps boost your immune system, supports digestion, and improves circulation, all of which contribute to your body's ability to prevent infections. Aim for a balanced exercise routine that includes cardiovascular workouts, strength training, and flexibility exercises like yoga or Pilates.

- Manage Stress: Stress is a known trigger for yeast infections because it can weaken your immune system and disrupt the balance of good bacteria in your body. Incorporating stress-relief practices such as meditation, deep breathing exercises, or mindfulness techniques can help reduce your risk of recurrent infections.

- Get Sufficient Sleep: Lack of sleep weakens the immune system, making it more difficult for your body to fight off infections. Prioritize restful sleep by maintaining a regular sleep schedule, creating a calming bedtime routine, and avoiding stimulants like caffeine late in the day.

Hydration and Skin Care

Staying hydrated is another simple yet effective way to rebuild your health after a yeast infection. Drinking plenty of water helps flush toxins from your body and supports the function of your organs, including your skin, which is often affected by yeast overgrowth.

- Hydration: Water helps maintain moisture balance in the body and supports overall health. Aim to drink at least 8 glasses of water a day, and avoid sugary drinks and excessive caffeine, which can contribute to dehydration.

- Skin Care: If your yeast infection affected your skin (e.g., in skin folds or areas prone to moisture), maintaining good hygiene is essential. Cleanse affected areas gently with mild, unscented soap and make sure they are completely dry before putting on clothes. Wearing breathable, moisture-wicking fabrics like cotton can also help prevent moisture buildup, which can trigger yeast growth.

Long-term Immune System Support

Your immune system is your first line of defense against infections, including yeast overgrowth. Strengthening it is key to preventing future episodes of infection. In addition to diet, exercise, and supplements, focusing on habits that promote a strong immune response will support long-term wellness.

- Limit Antibiotic Use: While antibiotics are necessary for treating bacterial infections, they can also disrupt your body's balance of good bacteria, leading to yeast overgrowth. When possible, avoid unnecessary antibiotics, and always discuss alternatives with your healthcare provider.

- Reduce Exposure to Environmental Toxins: Exposure to certain chemicals and toxins—whether through processed foods, personal care products, or environmental pollution—can weaken your immune system. Opt for natural, organic products when possible and minimize exposure to potential toxins by avoiding heavily processed foods, smoking, and excessive alcohol consumption.

- Stay Informed: Stay connected with your healthcare provider and keep yourself informed about new research, treatments, and strategies for maintaining health. Taking an active role in your healthcare will ensure that you're always making the best choices for your body.

Holistic Approach to Healing

Rebuilding your health after a yeast infection requires a holistic approach that considers not just physical recovery but also emotional well-being. Chronic or recurrent infections can be mentally draining, so incorporating self-care and mental wellness practices into your recovery is essential.

- Mind-Body Connection: Acknowledge the connection between your mental and physical health. Stress, anxiety, and emotional burnout can all contribute to physical illness, including yeast infections. Addressing emotional well-being through therapy, journaling, or relaxation techniques can help improve your overall health.

- Self-Care Routine: Create a daily self-care routine that includes time for relaxation, reflection, and mindfulness. Engaging in activities that bring you joy, whether it's reading, taking a walk, or practicing a hobby, can help reduce stress and improve your quality of life.

Chapter Four

How to Avoid Recurrent Yeast Infections

For many people, yeast infections can be a frustrating and recurrent issue. If you've experienced multiple infections, you're likely eager to find ways to break the cycle and prevent future outbreaks. Avoiding recurrent yeast infections requires a proactive approach that includes lifestyle adjustments, proper hygiene, and an understanding of the factors that trigger yeast overgrowth. Here's how to minimize the risk of future infections and maintain a healthy balance.

Understand the Triggers

The first step in preventing recurrent yeast infections is understanding what triggers them. Yeast infections occur when the fungus *Candida* grows out of control, which can be caused by various factors, such as:

- Antibiotic Use: Antibiotics can disrupt the balance of good bacteria in your body, allowing yeast to grow unchecked. If you need antibiotics, consider taking probiotics or eating fermented foods to help maintain your microbiome during and after treatment.

- Hormonal Changes: Hormonal fluctuations, such as those that occur during pregnancy, menstruation, or while taking birth control pills, can create an environment where yeast thrives. If you notice infections coinciding with hormonal changes, discuss alternative options with your healthcare provider.

- Diet High in Sugar and Refined Carbohydrates: Yeast feeds on sugar, so diets rich in sugar and processed foods can encourage yeast overgrowth. Reducing your sugar intake and incorporating more whole, nutrient-dense foods can help prevent infections.

- Stress and Lack of Sleep: Chronic stress and poor sleep weaken the immune system, making it easier for yeast to overgrow. Prioritizing rest and managing stress are crucial to keeping your body's natural defenses strong.

Improve Personal Hygiene and Habits

Your daily hygiene practices and habits can have a significant impact on whether or not you experience recurrent yeast infections. Small changes in how you care for your body can make a big difference in preventing yeast overgrowth.

- Wear Breathable, Loose-Fitting Clothing: Yeast thrives in warm, moist environments. Wearing tight clothing, especially synthetic fabrics, can trap heat and moisture, creating an ideal environment for yeast. Opt for loose-fitting clothing made from natural, breathable fabrics like cotton. This is especially important for underwear, workout clothes, and sleepwear.

- Change Out of Damp Clothing Promptly: After working out, swimming, or any activity that causes sweating, change out of damp clothing as soon as possible. Moisture from sweat or water can increase your risk of a yeast infection, especially in areas like the groin or under the breasts.

- Avoid Scented Products and Harsh Soaps: Scented soaps, feminine hygiene sprays, and douches can irritate the vaginal area and disrupt its natural balance. Use mild, unscented soaps to clean the area, and avoid douching, as it can remove beneficial bacteria that help prevent yeast overgrowth.

- Maintain Proper Vaginal Hygiene: Clean the vaginal area gently with water or mild soap, but avoid washing inside the vagina, as this can disturb the delicate balance of bacteria and yeast. Always wipe from front to back after using the bathroom to prevent the spread of bacteria that could lead to infection.

Adopt a Yeast-Preventing Diet

A healthy diet plays an essential role in maintaining the balance of good bacteria and yeast in your body. Making certain dietary adjustments can help prevent yeast infections from coming back.

- Reduce Sugar Intake: Since yeast feeds on sugar, cutting back on sugary foods like sweets, pastries, and sugary drinks can reduce the chances of yeast overgrowth. Limiting refined carbohydrates like white bread and pasta can also help.

- Increase Probiotic-Rich Foods: Probiotic foods like yogurt, kefir, kimchi, and sauerkraut contain beneficial bacteria that can help keep yeast levels in check. Including these foods in your diet can promote a healthy microbiome and protect against yeast infections.

- Focus on Anti-Inflammatory Foods: Foods rich in antioxidants and anti-inflammatory properties, such as leafy greens, berries, and fatty fish, can help support your immune system and reduce the risk of infections. Additionally, incorporating garlic, a natural antifungal, into your diet may help combat yeast overgrowth.

- Stay Hydrated: Drinking plenty of water supports your overall health and helps flush out toxins and excess yeast from your system. Proper hydration also aids digestion and prevents imbalances in your gut bacteria.

Manage Stress and Boost Immunity

Stress is a major factor that can weaken your immune system, making you more susceptible to yeast infections. Taking steps to reduce stress and strengthen your immune system can help prevent recurrent infections.

Practice Stress Management Techniques: Incorporating stress-relief practices like meditation, yoga, deep breathing exercises, or journaling can help you manage stress more effectively. Reducing stress not only improves your emotional well-being but also helps your immune system function optimally.

Get Enough Sleep: Adequate sleep is crucial for immune health. Aim for 7–9 hours of sleep per night to give your body the rest it needs to fight off infections and maintain a healthy balance.

· Exercise Regularly: Physical activity strengthens your immune system, improves circulation, and helps regulate hormones, all of which contribute to preventing yeast infections. Aim for at least 30 minutes of moderate exercise most days of the week.

- Support Your Immune System with Supplements: In addition to a healthy diet, you may consider supplements that support immune function and help prevent yeast infections. Vitamin C, vitamin D, zinc, and probiotics are all known to boost immune health and may reduce the risk of recurrent infections.

Be Mindful of Medications

Certain medications, particularly antibiotics and steroids, can disrupt the balance of bacteria in your body and lead to yeast infections. If you need to take these medications, talk to your healthcare provider about ways to minimize the impact on your microbiome.

- Probiotic Supplements During Antibiotic Treatment: If you're prescribed antibiotics, consider taking a probiotic supplement to help maintain the balance of good bacteria in your body. This can help prevent yeast overgrowth while you're taking the medication.

- Explore Alternative Treatments for Chronic Conditions: If you're frequently prescribed medications that trigger yeast infections, such as steroids or immunosuppressants, discuss alternative treatments with your doctor. They may be able to suggest options that are less likely to disrupt your body's balance.

Know When to Seek Medical Help

If you're experiencing recurrent yeast infections, it's important to consult with a healthcare professional to rule out underlying conditions that may be contributing to the problem. Conditions like diabetes, autoimmune disorders, or hormonal imbalances can make you more susceptible to yeast infections.

- Consult with a Specialist: If you've had multiple yeast infections in a short period, a gynecologist or infectious disease specialist can help determine the cause and develop a personalized treatment plan.

- Get Tested for Underlying Conditions: Conditions like diabetes or thyroid disorders can affect your body's ability to regulate yeast growth. If yeast infections persist despite your best efforts, testing for these conditions might reveal an underlying issue that needs to be addressed.

Long-Term Strategies for Prevention

Preventing yeast infections isn't about a one-time fix; it's about adopting long-term strategies to maintain a healthy balance in your body. By staying consistent with your hygiene, diet, and lifestyle choices, you can reduce the chances of recurrent infections.

- Stick to Preventative Habits: Incorporate these tips into your daily routine to create an environment where yeast is less likely to thrive. Regularly reassess your habits to ensure they're supporting your health and wellness.

- Stay Informed About Your Health: Continue to educate yourself about the causes and prevention of yeast infections. Regular check-ups with your healthcare provider and staying on top of any changes in your body can help you catch potential issues early and keep infections at bay.

Chapter Five

Sexual Health After Yeast Infections

Yeast infections can have a significant impact on your sexual health and intimacy. While these infections are not sexually transmitted, they can affect your comfort and confidence in sexual relationships. Understanding how yeast infections interact with sexual health, and knowing how to protect yourself and your partner, can help you regain confidence and comfort in your intimate life.

Understanding the Impact on Sexual Health

Yeast infections can cause discomfort and pain, making sex an uncomfortable or even painful experience during an active infection. Symptoms such as itching, burning, and swelling in the vaginal area (or penis in men) can significantly affect sexual desire and satisfaction. Even after symptoms subside, it may take time to feel comfortable resuming sexual activity.

- Physical Discomfort: Pain or discomfort during sex (dyspareunia) is a common complaint for those recovering from yeast infections. The inflammation and irritation caused by the infection can persist, even after the infection itself has cleared. It's important to listen to your body and avoid sexual activity until you're fully healed.

- Emotional and Mental Impact: Experiencing a yeast infection, especially recurrent infections, can take an emotional toll. Feelings of embarrassment, frustration, or anxiety about sexual health are ommon. It's important to address these emotions and communicate openly with your partner to reduce feelings of insecurity.

When to Resume Sexual Activity

Knowing when it's safe to resume sexual activity after a yeast infection is crucial to your recovery and overall sexual health. Engaging in sexual activity too soon can prolong healing or cause discomfort.

• Wait Until Symptoms Fully Subside: It's important to wait until all symptoms, including itching, burning, and swelling, have completely gone away before resuming sexual activity. Having sex too soon can irritate sensitive tissues and may increase the risk of reinfection.

• Be Aware of Lubrication Needs: After a yeast infection, the vaginal area may be drier than usual due to the healing process. Using a water-based, unscented lubricant during intercourse can help reduce friction and make sex more comfortable. Avoid lubricants with fragrances or chemicals that could irritate the area.

Communicating with Your Partner

Open communication with your partner is key to maintaining a healthy sexual relationship, especially after experiencing a yeast infection. Discussing your concerns, symptoms, and boundaries can help foster understanding and prevent discomfort or awkwardness during intimacy.

- Be Honest About Your Recovery: Let your partner know if you're not feeling ready to resume sexual activity. Explain that yeast infections can take time to fully heal, and that rushing into intimacy could cause pain or discomfort. A supportive partner will understand and prioritize your well-being.

- Discuss Preventative Measures: If you're prone to recurrent yeast infections, it may be helpful to discuss preventative strategies with your partner. This could include using condoms, maintaining good hygiene, and being mindful of sexual activity during periods of vulnerability (e.g., during hormonal changes or antibiotic use).

Protecting Your Partner

While yeast infections are not considered sexually transmitted infections (STIs), it is possible for partners to pass the infection back and forth, especially if they engage in sexual activity during an active infection. Taking precautions can help protect your partner and prevent reinfection.

- Use Condoms During Recovery: Using condoms during intercourse, especially after a recent infection, can reduce the risk of irritation and prevent the spread of yeast between partners. This is especially important if one partner is still experiencing symptoms or is prone to infections.

- Oral Sex Considerations: If either partner has an active yeast infection (including oral thrush), it's advisable to avoid oral sex until the infection has cleared. Oral yeast infections can be transmitted through oral-genital contact, leading to further discomfort or infection.

Rebuilding Confidence in Intimacy

Yeast infections can sometimes affect your confidence in sexual relationships. The discomfort and frustration caused by recurring infections may make you feel less attractive or desirable. However, it's important to remember that yeast infections are a common and treatable condition, and they do not define your worth or sexual desirability.

- Focus on Emotional Intimacy: If physical intimacy feels challenging after a yeast infection, focus on building emotional intimacy with your partner. Sharing your thoughts and feelings openly can strengthen your relationship and help you feel more connected.

- Take Your Time: There's no need to rush back into sexual activity. Take the time you need to heal both physically and emotionally. Building back your confidence in intimacy may take time, but going at your own pace will ensure you feel comfortable and in control of your body.

Preventing Yeast Infections from Impacting Future Intimacy

To reduce the likelihood of future yeast infections affecting your sexual health, consider adopting preventive strategies in your intimate life. Small changes can go a long way in maintaining a healthy balance and preventing recurrent infections.

- Maintain Good Hygiene: Before and after sexual activity, both partners should practice good hygiene to prevent the spread of bacteria or yeast. Washing the genital area with water or mild, unscented soap can help reduce the risk of irritation or infection.

- Choose the Right Contraceptives: Some contraceptives, such as diaphragms and spermicides, can disrupt the natural balance of bacteria in the vagina, potentially increasing the risk of yeast infections. If you're prone to infections, discuss alternative methods of contraception with your healthcare provider.

- Use Breathable Fabrics: Wearing breathable underwear made from cotton can help reduce moisture buildup, which creates an environment where yeast thrives. This is especially important after sexual activity, when moisture levels may increase.

Seeking Professional Support

If yeast infections are consistently affecting your sexual health and relationships, don't hesitate to seek professional support. A gynecologist or sexual health specialist can help you address the root causes of recurring infections and provide guidance on how to maintain a healthy sex life.

Sexual Health Counseling: If yeast infections are causing emotional or relational strain, a sexual health counselor or therapist can help you and your partner navigate these challenges. They can offer strategies for rebuilding confidence and communication in your intimate life.

Medical Advice: If you experience recurrent yeast infections, it may be helpful to undergo a medical evaluation to determine if there are underlying issues contributing to the infections. Your healthcare provider can recommend treatment options, including antifungal medications, probiotics, or lifestyle changes to help prevent future infections.

Chapter Six

Developing a Long-Term Care Plan

For those who experience recurrent yeast infections, a long-term care plan is essential for maintaining overall health and preventing future outbreaks. A well-thought-out care plan focuses on managing risk factors, supporting the immune system, and taking proactive steps to balance the body's natural defenses. This chapter will guide you in creating a sustainable approach to managing and preventing yeast infections over the long term.

Understanding the Need for a Long-Term Care Plan

Recurrent yeast infections can be a sign that something in your lifestyle, health, or environment is continuously triggering these episodes. A long-term care plan addresses the root causes of yeast infections rather than just treating the symptoms. By developing a sustainable plan, you can reduce the frequency of infections and support your body's natural balance.

A long-term care plan should address:
- Identifying triggers that contribute to yeast overgrowth.
- Prevention strategies for managing diet, hygiene, and other factors.
- Ongoing support for immune health, hormonal balance, and mental well-being.

Assessing Your Risk Factors

The first step in developing a long-term care plan is identifying the factors that increase your risk of yeast infections. Understanding your personal triggers allows you to focus on areas where you can make changes to minimize future infections.

- Medical History: Certain medical conditions, such as diabetes or autoimmune disorders, can increase your susceptibility to yeast infections. If you have an underlying condition, work with your healthcare provider to manage it and monitor how it affects your risk of infections.

- Medications: Long-term use of antibiotics, corticosteroids, or hormonal treatments (like birth control pills) can disrupt your body's balance and lead to recurrent infections. Discuss alternative medications or preventive measures with your doctor if these treatments are necessary for your health.

- Lifestyle and Hygiene: Assessing your daily habits is key to identifying potential triggers. Factors such as wearing tight clothing, using scented products, or consuming a high-sugar diet can increase your risk of infections.

Establishing Healthy Habits for Prevention

A successful long-term care plan is built on a foundation of healthy habits that support your body's natural ability to prevent yeast overgrowth. These habits should become part of your daily routine to ensure lasting results.

- Maintain a Balanced Diet: Diet plays a central role in preventing yeast infections. Focus on limiting sugar and refined carbohydrates, which feed yeast, while incorporating probiotic-rich foods to support your gut health. Consistent hydration is also crucial to keeping your system balanced and flushing out excess yeast.

- Practice Good Hygiene: Simple adjustments to your hygiene routine can help prevent recurrent infections. Wash with mild, unscented soaps, avoid douching, and wear breathable fabrics to keep moisture at bay. It's also important to change out of wet clothing, like swimsuits or gym clothes, as soon as possible.

- Support Your Immune System: A healthy immune system is your first line of defense against yeast infections. Regular exercise, proper sleep, and stress management are all key components of a strong immune system. Consider supplementing your diet with vitamins like C, D, and zinc to further boost your immunity.

Hormonal Balance and Yeast Infections

Hormonal fluctuations, such as those that occur during menstruation, pregnancy, or while using birth control, can trigger yeast infections. If hormonal imbalances are contributing to your yeast infections, addressing these fluctuations can be an essential part of your long-term care plan.

- Natural Hormonal Support: If you're experiencing hormonal imbalances, discuss natural solutions with your healthcare provider. Certain lifestyle changes, such as reducing stress, eating hormoneupportive foods (like flaxseeds or leafy greens), nd staying physically active, can help stabilize your ormones.

Hormone Therapy Alternatives: If birth control or ormone replacement therapy is contributing to our yeast infections, you may want to explore lternative forms of contraception or hormone management. Speak with your healthcare provider bout options that are less likely to disrupt your ody's balance.

Managing Stress and Mental Well-Being

Chronic stress can weaken your immune system, making you more vulnerable to infections, including yeast infections. Developing a strategy for managing stress is a crucial part of your long-term care plan. Additionally, emotional well-being is important for handling the frustrations that often accompany recurrent infections.

- Stress-Relief Techniques: Incorporating stress management techniques into your daily life can reduce your overall stress levels and boost your immune system. Practices such as meditation, deep breathing exercises, yoga, and mindfulness are excellent ways to keep stress in check.

- Seeking Emotional Support: Dealing with recurrent yeast infections can be emotionally draining. Don't hesitate to seek support from a therapist or counselor if you're struggling to manage the mental toll. Joining a support group or speaking openly with friends and family can also help reduce the emotional burden.

Working with Healthcare Providers

Collaborating with your healthcare provider is essential in developing an effective long-term care plan. Your doctor can help you identify underlying causes, suggest treatments, and provide guidance on preventive strategies.

- Regular Check-Ups: If you're prone to recurrent yeast infections, schedule regular check-ups with your doctor or gynecologist. Ongoing monitoring can help you catch any infections early and adjust your care plan as needed.

- Customized Treatment Plans: In some cases, recurrent yeast infections may require customized treatment options. Your doctor may recommend long-term antifungal treatments, probiotics, or other interventions to help manage your condition. They can also help you explore natural or alternative treatments if you prefer a holistic approach.

Monitoring Your Progress

Your long-term care plan is not static—it should evolve as your body and lifestyle change. Monitoring your progress allows you to assess whether your prevention strategies are working and make adjustments as necessary.

- Keep a Health Journal: Track your diet, stress levels, symptoms, and any potential triggers in a health journal. This can help you identify patterns and pinpoint what's working or what might need adjustment.

- Stay Flexible: Your care plan should adapt to changes in your life, health, and environment. If you find that certain strategies are no longer effective, don't hesitate to adjust them or consult your healthcare provider for further guidance.

Building a Support Network

Having a support network can make a big difference in managing recurrent yeast infections over the long term. Whether it's through friends, family, healthcare providers, or support groups, having people to lean on will help you stay committed to your care plan and feel less isolated.

- Lean on Loved Ones: Don't hesitate to talk to your loved ones about your condition. While yeast nfections can feel like a private issue, having emotional support can alleviate stress and help you stay on track with your care plan.

· Join Support Groups: Online or in-person support groups for those dealing with chronic infections can provide a sense of community and shared experience. Learning from others' experiences and sharing your own struggles can be comforting and empowering.

Chapter Seven

How Menopause and Birth Control Impact Infections

Hormonal changes play a significant role in the body's susceptibility to yeast infections, especially for women. Two major factors that can disrupt hormonal balance and contribute to recurring yeast infections are menopause and the use of hormonal birth control. Understanding how these hormonal shifts impact your body is crucial in managing and preventing infections.

Menopause and Yeast Infections

Menopause marks a significant change in a woman's life, characterized by a natural decline in estrogen levels. This hormonal shift can have a profound effect on vaginal health and yeast balance, increasing the likelihood of infections.

Declining Estrogen Levels: Estrogen plays an important role in maintaining vaginal health by supporting the production of healthy vaginal flora (good bacteria) and maintaining the natural acidity of the vaginal environment. As estrogen levels drop during menopause, the vaginal tissue can become thinner, drier, and less acidic. This change in the vaginal environment can lead to an overgrowth of yeast, increasing the risk of infections.

Vaginal Dryness and pH Changes: During menopause, many women experience vaginal dryness and changes in the vaginal pH balance, making it easier for yeast to thrive. With less moisture and fewer healthy bacteria to keep yeast in check, the risk of developing recurrent yeast infections increases.

· Weakening of Vaginal Tissues: As estrogen levels drop, vaginal tissues may weaken, making them more susceptible to irritation and infection. This weakening can result in increased discomfort during sexual activity, and a higher risk of infections, including yeast infections.

How to Manage Yeast Infections During Menopause

Managing yeast infections during menopause requires addressing the hormonal changes that affect vaginal health. Here are some strategies:

- Vaginal Moisturizers: Using vaginal moisturizers or lubricants can help alleviate dryness and reduce irritation. Opt for unscented, water-based products that won't disrupt the vaginal pH.

- Hormone Replacement Therapy (HRT): For some women, hormone replacement therapy can help restore estrogen levels and improve vaginal health. Topical estrogen creams or vaginal rings can specifically target the vaginal area, helping to maintain healthy tissue and reduce the risk of infections. Consult with your healthcare provider to see if HRT is appropriate for you.

- Probiotics: Taking probiotics or using probiotic vaginal suppositories can help restore the balance of good bacteria in the vaginal environment. This can help prevent yeast overgrowth and maintain a healthy vaginal microbiome.

- Diet and Lifestyle Changes: Adopting a diet rich in phytoestrogens (plant-based estrogens), such as flaxseeds, soy, and legumes, may help support hormone balance. Regular exercise and stress management are also important for overall well-being and hormone regulation during menopause.

Hormonal Birth Control and Yeast Infections

Hormonal birth control methods, such as birth control pills, patches, and intrauterine devices (IUDs), can also impact yeast infections by altering hormone levels in the body. The synthetic hormones in these contraceptives can influence the balance of bacteria and yeast in the vagina, leading to a higher risk of infections for some women.

- Estrogen and Progesterone Effects: Hormonal birth control methods often contain synthetic versions of estrogen and progesterone. These hormones can affect the natural balance of yeast and bacteria in the body, sometimes leading to an overgrowth of *Candida*, the fungus responsible for yeast infections. Estrogen, in particular, can cause the vaginal lining to produce more glycogen, a type of sugar, which provides fuel for yeast to grow.

- Impact on Vaginal pH: Birth control methods that alter hormone levels may also impact the vaginal pH, making it less acidic and more prone to yeast overgrowth. A healthy vaginal pH is typically slightly acidic, which helps control the growth of yeast. When this balance is disrupted by hormonal changes, the likelihood of infection increases.

How to Manage Yeast Infections While Using Birth Control

f you are experiencing recurrent yeast infections while using hormonal birth control, there are several options to consider:

- Switching Birth Control Methods: If you suspect that your birth control method is contributing to recurrent infections, consider discussing alternative options with your healthcare provider. Non-hormonal options, such as copper IUDs, condoms, or fertility awareness methods, may reduce the risk of yeast infections by not interfering with hormone levels.

- Taking Probiotics: Just like during menopause, probiotics can help maintain the balance of good bacteria in your body and reduce the risk of yeast overgrowth. You can incorporate probiotic supplements or foods like yogurt, kefir, and sauerkraut into your daily routine.

- Support Vaginal Health: Maintaining good hygiene, wearing breathable underwear, and avoiding tight clothing can help prevent yeast infections while on birth control. In addition, using mild, unscented cleansers for vaginal hygiene can reduce irritation

Comparing Menopause and Birth Control Effects on Yeast Infections

Although menopause and birth control both involve hormonal changes, the effects on yeast infections differ based on the underlying hormonal shifts.

- Menopause: The decrease in estrogen during menopause leads to vaginal dryness, thinning tissues, and a less acidic environment, all of which can contribute to yeast infections.

- Birth Control: Hormonal birth control introduces synthetic hormones that may increase the production of glycogen in the vagina, providing a food source for yeast and potentially disrupting the vaginal microbiome.

Both scenarios highlight the importance of hormone balance in maintaining vaginal health and preventing infections. Whether you're dealing with he hormonal changes of menopause or the effects f birth control, understanding these connections llows you to make informed decisions about your ealth and develop effective strategies to prevent east infections.

Seeking Professional Advice

f you're experiencing recurrent yeast infections lue to menopause or hormonal birth control, it's mportant to seek medical advice. A healthcare orovider can help determine the best course of iction based on your individual circumstances and nedical history.

- Menopause Care: If yeast infections are a frequent ssue during menopause, talk to your doctor about reatments such as hormone replacement therapy or non-hormonal interventions to improve vaginal iealth.

- Birth Control Adjustments: If hormonal birth control seems to be the cause of recurrent infections, your doctor can help you explore alternative contraceptive options that might better suit your body's needs.

Chapter Eight

Thriving Post-Infection: Mindset Shifts

After dealing with a yeast infection, especially if it's recurrent, it's not just your body that needs healing—your mindset plays a critical role in how you move forward. It's easy to get trapped in frustration, fear, or embarrassment, but shifting your mindset can help you reclaim your sense of well-being, confidence, and control. This chapter explores how adopting new perspectives and mental strategies can help you thrive after a yeast infection.

Moving from Frustration to Empowerment

Repeated infections can leave you feeling helpless or defeated, but it's important to recognize that you have the power to take control of your health. Instead of viewing yeast infections as an ongoing battle you can't win, shift your mindset toward empowerment. This means acknowledging the things within your control, like lifestyle choices, hygiene practices, and diet, and using this knowledge to prevent future infections.

- Educate Yourself: Knowledge is power. The more you understand about what causes yeast infections, the better equipped you'll be to prevent them. Take the time to learn about your body's signals, triggers, and the ways you can protect yourself. Feeling informed can replace frustration with confidence.

- Take Ownership of Your Health: Rather than seeing yeast infections as something that happens *to* you, start viewing yourself as an active participant in your own health journey. This mindset shift can help you feel more in control and less like a victim of recurring infections.

Letting Go of Shame

One of the most harmful mindsets that can follow a yeast infection is shame. Many people feel embarrassed or uncomfortable talking about these infections, even though they are incredibly common. Letting go of this shame is a crucial step in thriving post-infection.

- Normalize Your Experience: Yeast infections are a medical condition, not a reflection of your cleanliness or personal worth. Remind yourself that millions of people experience them every year, and there's nothing to be ashamed of. Talking openly with a trusted friend or loved one can also help reduce feelings of shame.

- *Shift Your Focus to Healing Instead of fixating on the discomfort or embarrassment of an infection, shift your focus to the steps you can take to heal. Prioritizing your recovery and well-being can help you let go of any negative self-talk or shame you may be experiencing.

From Fear to Confidence

If you've dealt with recurrent infections, it's normal to fear the next one. However, living in fear of another outbreak can affect your mental health and limit your sense of freedom. Shifting from fear to confidence involves trusting in your ability to manage your health and prevent future infections.

- Trust Your Plan: If you've developed a long-term care plan to prevent yeast infections, trust in it. By following healthy habits, managing stress, and maintaining good hygiene, you can reduce the likelihood of future infections. Building confidence in your routine will ease the fear of recurrence.

- Accept Uncertainty: It's important to acknowledge that despite your best efforts, you might experience another infection. However, this doesn't mean you've failed. Accepting the uncertainty while maintaining a positive outlook on prevention can reduce anxiety and help you remain resilient.

Reclaiming Body Confidence

Yeast infections can make you feel disconnected from your body, especially if they've affected your sexual health or daily comfort. Reclaiming your body confidence is an essential part of thriving post-infection.

Celebrate Your Body's Resilience: Instead of focusing on what went wrong, acknowledge how your body has healed. Your body is resilient and capable of recovering from infections. Celebrate the fact that you're taking care of yourself and doing what's necessary to maintain your health.

Focus on Self-Care: Practicing self-care rituals can help you reconnect with your body and build confidence. Whether it's through skincare, exercise, meditation, or relaxation, nurturing your body will help you feel more positive and in tune with yourself.

Embracing Patience and Self-Compassion

Recovery, both physical and emotional, takes time. Adopting a mindset of patience and self-compassion can help you manage the stress that sometimes follows an infection.

- Give Yourself Time to Heal: Healing is a process, and it's important to be patient with yourself as you recover. Whether it's physical symptoms that take time to subside or emotional discomfort lingering after recurrent infections, remind yourself that recovery doesn't happen overnight.

- Practice Self-Compassion: Be kind to yourself throughout the process. It's easy to be self-critical when dealing with health challenges, but self-compassion is key to emotional recovery. Treat yourself with the same understanding and care that you would offer to a friend in a similar situation.

Looking Ahead with Optimism

The experience of dealing with yeast infections can be overwhelming, but it doesn't have to define your future. Shifting your mindset toward optimism allows you to focus on the positive steps you've taken and the healthier future you're working toward.

- Focus on What You've Learned: Every experience, including dealing with yeast infections, teaches you something about your body and health. Take what you've learned about prevention, care, and your own personal needs, and use that knowledge to build a healthier future.

- Visualize a Positive Future: Instead of worrying about the next infection, visualize yourself thriving in the future. Imagine yourself healthy, confident, and in control of your well-being. This optimistic outlook will help guide your actions and keep you motivated to stick with your long-term care plan.

Surround Yourself with Support

Having a support network can help reinforce your mindset shifts and encourage positive thinking. Whether it's friends, family, or healthcare professionals, surrounding yourself with people who support your health journey is vital to thriving post-infection.

- Lean on Trusted Individuals: Don't hesitate to talk about your experiences with those you trust. Sharing your journey can provide emotional relief and help you feel less isolated in dealing with yeast infections.

- Seek Professional Guidance: If recurring infections are affecting your mental health, consider seeking guidance from a therapist or counselor. A mental health professional can help you work through any feelings of anxiety, fear, or frustration related to your condition.